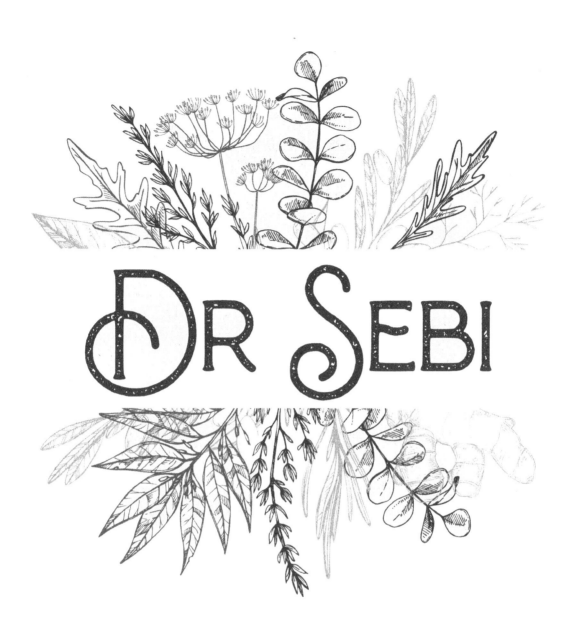

Dr Sebi

A Complete Beginner's Guide to the Alkaline Diet. Learn About Dr. Sebi's philosophy, How to Detoxify Your Body, Get Rid of Mucus and Stop Inflammations

Joseph Meyer

Sommary

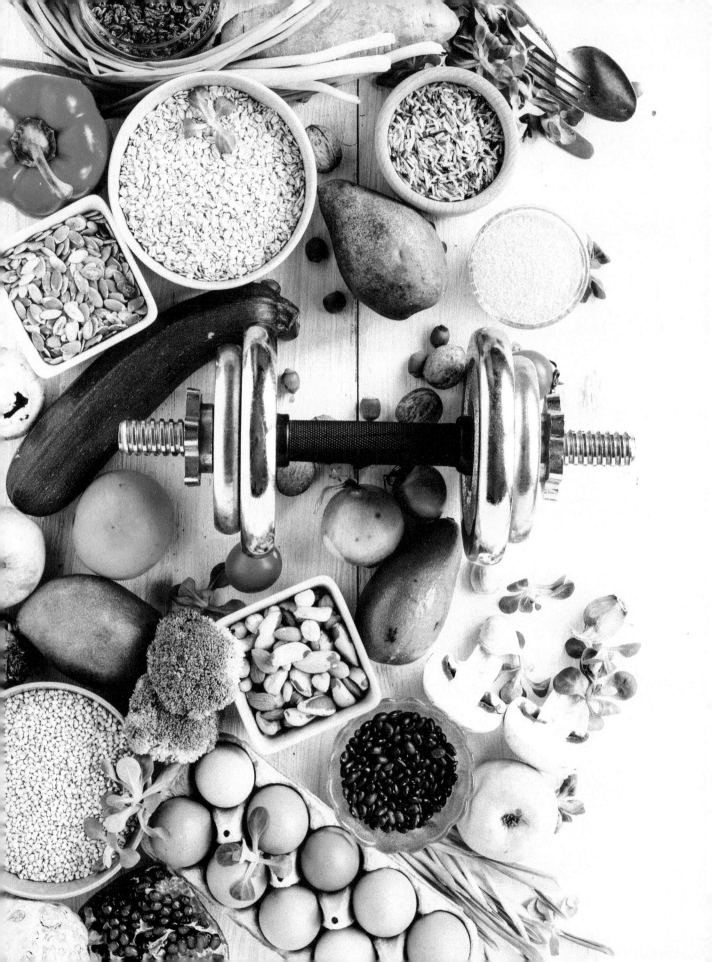

Introduction

The technique introduced by Dr. Sebi was effective in eradicating illnesses. Diseases are a consequence of the host being contaminated by a germ, virus, or bacteria, according to Western medical science. Inorganic, carcinogenic compounds are used in their approach to handling these infestations. On the opposite, by simple deductive logic, Dr. Sebi's study instantly uncovers inconsistencies in their premise. They also repeatedly yielded unsuccessful outcomes while repeatedly using the same premise and techniques. In essence, their approach to disease care has failed to deliver any cures in the 400-year history of the European philosophy of medicine.

Natural plants contain the African Bio-Mineral Balance compounds; this suggests that their structure is alkaline in nature. This is significant and influential in the progress of Dr. Sebi in correcting pathologies—since illness may only occur in an acid-based environment; thus, when handling illness, it is contradictory to use inorganic compounds because they are acid-based. A diseased body can be successfully washed and detoxified only through consistent usage of natural botanical treatments, reversing it to its expected alkaline condition.

Dr. Sebi's diet scheme goes much better. The African Bio-Mineral Balance absorbs degraded minerals and rejuvenates weakened cell tissue eroded by the acid, diseased state, in addition to eliminating the buildup of years of toxins. The scalp, intestine, gall bladder, lymph glands, kidneys, and the colon are the main organs of expulsion. If all contaminants are extracted from the above-mentioned tissues, they can be recycled, manifesting disease in the whole body. In the poorest tissues, the body gradually breaks down owing to the failure to dissipate the effects of contaminants. The colon is the most critical organ that must be cleansed before any illness can be reversed by detoxifying. The other main organs will be left toxic if the colon is the only organ cleansed and detoxified, thereby leaving the disease in the body.

The plant-based diet formulated by the late Dr. Sebi is called the "Dr. Sebi's diet," sometimes named the "Dr. Sebi's Alkaline diet." By alkalizing your blood, it rejuvenates your cells by removing radioactive waste. The diet depends, along with several nutrients, on consuming a limited list of permitted foods. This diet is focused on the principle of African Bio-Mineral Equilibrium and was developed by Alfredo Darrington Bowman, a self-educated herbalist best known as Dr. Sebi. Without focusing on traditional Western medicine, he developed this diet for everyone who wants to spontaneously treat or avoid sickness and enhance their general well-being. You would find it highly helpful and efficient to recover the normal alkaline condition of your body and detoxify your diseased body by solely observing his lifestyle and utilizing his supplements. The advantages of Dr. Sebi's diet and how empirical research supports its health statements would be mentioned in this book.

Chapter 1

Know About Alkaline and Acid Metabolism

Metabolism is a chemical reaction that happens in the cells of the body that converts food into energy. Our bodies use this power to do everything from moving to learning to creating. Relevant proteins inside the body activate the chemical processes of Metabolism. Hundreds of biochemical reactions exist at the same time, all regulated by the body, to keep the cells healthy and functional.

1.1 KNOWING ABOUT WORKING OF METABOLISM
The digestive system utilizes enzymes when we consume food in order to:
- Break down proteins into amino acids.
- Convert fats into fatty acids.
- Transform carbohydrates into basic sugars (glucose, for instance).

The body can use amino acids, sugar, and fatty acids as sources of energy when necessary. These compounds are absorbed in the blood, which brings them to the tissues. Once they enter the cells, other enzymes serve to speed up or track the chemical processes connected with the "metabolization" of these compounds. Throughout these phases, the energy from such compounds is released for the body to use or gets stored in the body tissues, especially in the muscles, liver, and body fat. A Metabolism is a balancing act involving two concurrently occurring modes of events:

- **Anabolism:** Anabolism, or positive Metabolism, is all about creating and maintaining. Throughout the process, body cells are built up, and energy is stored. It encourages the new creation of cells, protection of body tissue, and storage of resources for future use. In Anabolism, small molecules turn into broader, more complex glucose, fat molecules, and proteins.

•   **Catabolism:** Destructive Metabolism or Catabolism is the process that produces the energy required for any activity in the cells. It involves the breakdown of body tissues and the resulting storage of energy to gain more energy for body functions. Cells break down the big molecules (mainly fats and carbohydrates) to generate energy. This offers fuel for Anabolism, heating up the body, which allows the muscles to contract, and carries the body.

As complex chemical units break down into more essential compounds, the body creates waste products from the skin, kidneys, lungs, and intestines.

1.2 HOW IS METABOLISM CONTROLLED?

Different hormones of the endocrine system help control the metabolism speed and course. In determining how fast or steadily is the chemical metabolism processes in the body of a person, a thyroid gland-made, released hormone, thyroxine, plays a key part. The organ, pancreas, secretes hormones that help to determine at any point if the body's key metabolic role is anabolic or catabolic. For instance, more anabolic activity usually happens while a person eats a meal. That's how eating raises the volume of glucose in the blood. The pancreas senses this high glucose amount and stimulates insulin, the hormone, which signals cells to increase their anabolic activities.

Metabolism is a complex chemical system. So, it's no wonder that a lot of individuals think of it in the simplest form: as something that dictates how easily the body gain or lose weight. This is where the calories gather. A calorie is a unit which decides how much energy a specific meal gives to a body. A bar of chocolate produces more calories than an avocado, so it supplies the body with more energy, although sometimes too many calories aren't a good thing. As the car retains fuel in the gas tank until it is required to run the engine, the body retains calories, specifically as fat. When one overfills a car's gas tank, it leaks over onto the pavement. Likewise, when a person eats so many calories, they turn out in the form of extra body fat. How well the person workouts, the amount of muscle and fat in his body, and the person's basal metabolic rate (BMR) affect the calories that anyone burns each day. BMR is a measure of the rate at which a body "burns" fat in the form of calories while at rest.

BMR can play an important role in an individual's tendency to gain weight. E.g., anyone with a low BMR will tend to gain more body fat over some time than an individual with a normal BMR of similar size who eats the exact amount of food and does the exact amount of exercise, and therefore consumes fewer calories while sleeping or sitting.

BMR can be defined by an individual's genes and by some health conditions. The composition of the body also induces it; individuals with more muscles and less fat usually have higher BMRs. People will change their BMR in certain situations. For example, a person who exercises more does not only lose more calories but often becomes physically stronger, improving his BMR.

1.3 BLOOD'S FUNCTION IN METABOLISM SUPPORT

A person cannot survive without blood, and the heart is pumping the blood through the body's vast network of arteries and veins, supplying oxygen to cells. Blood is a circulatory system that transfers consumed nutrients to the cells, such as amino acids, O2, and oxygen, to waste products from cells such as CO_2 and urea to kidneys.

It promotes cellular Metabolism by transferring waste materials and macromolecules that are synthesized. In essence, chemicals are exchanged, such as hormones, facilitating communication between organs. The volume of blood that circulates is about 5 liters in the adult human body, which provides for about 8% of the human body's weight.

How Blood Substances Support Blood Function?

Blood is almost 78% liquid and 22% solid by volume. The liquid is Plasma and primarily the water portion of the blood (95%), but it also contains proteins such as lipoproteins, albumin, ions, amino acids, oxygen, lipids, minerals, carbohydrates, waste materials from ammonia and hormones, urea, enzymes, and gases. The albumin protein is found in the blood in insignificant quantities. Albumin appears to preserve the balance of fluid between tissue and blood, and it helps to keep a steady blood pH. The liquid component of the blood is important for the activities as a transportation vessel, and thus the electrolytes contained in the blood maintain a steady pH and fluid balance. Besides, the large content of blood water helps to sustain body temperature and constant flow of blood distributors. The blood is particularly good at regulating temperature, so even when it reaches the lungs to the nose, it works as a regulator by warming the cool air through the nose's small blood vessels.

Nutrients
Nutrients continue to be transferred from the small intestine to cells before they are swallowed. Moreover, molecules that are generated in many other cells also need to be transferred to other organs. The channel is blood, and blood vessels distribute nutrients and molecules to all cells. Like certain carbohydrates, minerals, fats, and some proteins, water-soluble substances migrate through the blood independently. Triglycerides, fat-soluble vitamins, cholesterol, and other lipids are packaged into lipoproteins that allow the transportation of blood in a watery environment. Several proteins, medicines, and hormones, especially albumin, are based on transport carriers. As well as transporting all of these molecules, blood would pass the breathed in oxygen by the lungs to all cells in the body. This is accomplished by the hemoglobin, an iron-containing molecule in the red blood cells.

Wastes Out
Cells contain water and carbon dioxide as surplus products in the energy metabolism of macronutrients. When blood flows through narrower and fewer channels, the blood flow volume is dramatically reduced, causing cellular waste products to be quickly substituted for nutrients and oxygen. The kidneys eliminate any remaining water in the blood, and blood carries CO_2 to the lungs where it is breathed out. The liver also creates the waste product as urea from the degradation of amino acids and detoxifies several toxic compounds, all of which involve kidney excretion from the blood.

1.4 INTERCONNECTIVITY BETWEEN ORGAN SYSTEMS
The organ systems in the human body rely on each other for continued survival as a complex system. Blood provides for the movement of nutrients, waste, heat, fluids, and is often a conduit for interaction with organ systems. The concept of blood to the rest of the body is accurately presented in its role in the delivery of glucose, particularly to the brain. Per hour, the brain regulates 6 grams of glucose in total. To prevent confusion, stroke, and even death, glucose must be readily available to the brain at all times. To fulfill this task, cells in the

pancreas sense glucose levels in the blood. If glucose levels are inadequate, the glucagon hormone is released into the blood and is transported to the liver, where it transmits the signal to produce glycogen breakdown and glucose output. Since glucose is absorbed in the blood and brings it to the brain, this is just what the liver does. Oxygen is supplied by blood at the same time to facilitate brain energy from the Metabolism of glucose. Healthy blood performs its tasks successfully, avoiding collapse and death from hypoglycemia.

1.5 WHAT MAKES BLOOD HEALTHY?

It is important to conserve healthy blood, including its continuous recycling, to ensure its wide variety of essential functions. Blood is durable because it comprises sufficient quantities of cellular components and water; the concentration of dissolved substances such as albumin and electrolytes are sufficient. Blood has to function optimally for micro and macronutrients, along with all other tissues. A large amount of hemoglobin loaded into each red blood cell, with the other enzymes, cellular organelles, must be generated by amino acids where blood cells are made in the bone marrow. Red blood cells utilize glucose as oxygen, similarly to the brain, and it must stay in constant supply to maintain red blood cell synthesis. As in many other species, blood cells are surrounded by a plasma membrane, which is primarily composed of lipids.

1.6 WHAT CAN BLOOD TESTS TELL YOU ABOUT YOUR HEALTH?

Blood is the source of biomolecular materials and wastes; through analyzing the blood components and particular substances present in the blood, not just the state of the blood, but often the health of other organ systems can be revealed. In regular blood checks administered at the annual medical examination, the usual blood tests done will warn the doctor regarding the functioning of a particular organ or about the risk of cancer.

A biomarker is defined as a molecule or function observable that is related to a specific disease or health condition. Biomarker levels in the blood are indicative of the likelihood of disease; some biomarkers are insulin, triglycerides, prostate-specific antigens, and cholesterol. Blood examination results include the concentrations of substances in a person's blood that display the normal distributions for a given population category. Many variables can influence a person's blood test levels and cause them to fall under the normal range, such as the level of physical activity, diet, consumption of alcohol, and intake of medicine, but the results of blood tests below the "usual" range are not generally predictive of health problems. Measuring different blood factors allows us to diagnose the risk of disease and is indicative of the overall state of health.

1.7 CRITICAL FUNCTION OF BLOOD IS TO REGULATE PH: ACIDITY AND ALKALINITY

An integral property of the blood is the degree of alkalinity and acidity. On the pH scale, for blood, the acidity or alkalinity can be seen. The pH scale goes from zero (highly acidic) to 14 (basic or highly alkaline). The 7.0 pH of the scale is known as neutral. Blood is typically moderately basic, with a standard pH range of around 7.35–7.45. Usually, the body maintains a blood pH of close to 7.40.

A physician measures the acid-base equilibrium of a patient by measuring the pH and concentrations of bicarbonate (a base) and carbon dioxide (an acid) in the blood.

In the blood, the acidity rises when:

- Increases in the volume of acidic compounds in the body (through improved absorption or production or decreased elimination).
- Decreases in the body's volume of basic (alkaline) substances (through decreased intake or production or increased removal).
- As the level of acidity of the body decreases or as the base level increases, the blood alkalinity changes.

Control of Acid-Base Balance

Acid-Base Balance is characterized as the balance of the body's acidity and alkalinity. As many organs can be severely affected by such a slight deviation from the normal range, the base-acid balance of the blood is specifically controlled. To control the acid-base composition of the blood, the body utilizes distinct pathways. Such procedures require the stage of:

1. **The lungs:** One mechanism that the body uses to control blood pH is the release of carbon dioxide from the lungs. Moderately acidic carbon dioxide is a product of oxygen and nutrient absorption (Metabolism) (it is done by all cells) and, as such, is constantly created by cells. CO_2 then runs from the cells in the blood. Blood takes carbon dioxide to the lungs. From there, it is breathed out. As carbon dioxide builds up in the bloodstream, the pH of the

blood decreases, and acidity increases in the blood.

2. The brain regulates the carbon dioxide that is needed to be exhaled by controlling the velocity and rate of breathing (ventilation). The amount of carbon dioxide exhaled increases as respiration becomes stronger and deeper, and thus the pH of the blood. By adjusting the speed and rate of breathing, the lungs and brain are able to regulate the blood pH moment by moment.

3. **The kidneys:** The kidney's effects are by having some ability to adjust the amount of excreted acid or base, but this adjustment usually takes several days as the kidneys make these changes more gradually than the lungs do.

4. **Buffer system:** Another mechanism for managing blood pH is also the use of chemical buffer mechanisms that defend against sudden shifts in alkalinity and acidity. The pH buffer mechanisms are the normally existing variations of weak acids and weak bases in the body. The weak bases and acids exist in pairs that are in equilibrium under normal pH conditions. The pH buffer systems act chemically to counteract changes to the pH of a solution by adjusting the proportion of base and acid.

Among the most critical pH buffer systems in the blood are carbonic acid (a light acid formed by dissolving carbon dioxide in the blood) and bicarbonate ions (the corresponding weak base).

1.8 TYPES OF ACID-BASE DISORDERS

There are two acid-base composition abnormalities:

- **Acidosis:** There is too much acid (or very little base) in the blood, which contributes to a drop in blood pH.
- **Alkalosis:** There is too much base (or very little acid) in the blood, which results in a pH rise in the blood.

Alkalosis and acidosis are not considered to be pathogens, but the wide range of disorders is the result of these factors. For doctors, the occurrence of acidosis or alkalosis provides a vital sign that there is a serious problem.

Types of Alkalosis and Acidosis

Based upon their primary source, acidosis and alkalosis are categorized as: Metabolic and Respiratory.

- Metabolic alkalosis and metabolic acidosis are triggered by an excess of the production or excretion of acids or bases by the kidneys.

• Respiratory alkalosis and pulmonary acidosis cause shifts in carbon dioxide exhalation due to lung or breathing disorders. There could be more than one acid-base disorder in people.

Acid-Base Disorders Compensation

Each acid-base disturbance causes automatic compensatory processes that push the blood's pH back to normal. In addition, the respiratory system compensates for disturbances of metabolic, while physiological mechanisms compensate for disruptions of respiratory.

The compensatory processes would initially return the pH to close to nature. Therefore, if the blood pH has risen significantly, it indicates that the body's ability to compensate is insufficient. Doctors, in such cases, desperately search for and treat the underlying cause of the acid-base malfunction.

What Is Acidosis?

It's called acidosis if the fluids in the body contain too much acid. Acidosis develops when the lungs and kidneys cannot keep the body's pH in balance. Many of the body's functions produce acid. The kidneys and lungs will usually account for minor pH imbalances, but problems with these organs can contribute to the body storing excess acid.

The acidity of the blood is determined by measuring its pH. A lower pH shows that the blood is more acidic, and a higher pH shows that the blood is more basic. The pH should be about 7.4 in the blood. As per the American Association, acidosis is classified as a pH of 7.35 or below. A 7.45 or higher pH standard describes alkalosis. While seemingly insignificant, these numerical differences can be serious. Acidosis can lead to several health problems and can cause life-threatening situations.

Causes of Acidosis

There are two types of acidosis, both with distinct reasons. The type of acidosis is classified as either metabolic acidosis and lung acidosis, based on the prevalent cause of acidosis.

Respiratory Acidosis

Respiratory acidosis occurs in the body because of too many CO_2 stores. When a person is breathing, the lungs normally extract CO_2. The body can't always get rid of sufficiently CO_2, though. This can happen due to:

- Severe airway problems like hypertension.
- A chest injury.
- Obesity, which makes it hard to breathe.
- Misuse of sedatives.
- Overuse of liquor.
- A weakness of the muscles in the chest.
- Nervous system issues.
- Deformed chest structure.

Metabolic Acidosis

Metabolic acidosis starts in the kidneys, not in the lungs. It occurs when they are unable to remove sufficient acid or if they excrete out of too much base. Metabolic acidosis occurs in four primary forms:

- Acidosis in diabetics: This arises in persons with badly managed diabetes. In the circulation, ketones build up and acidify the blood if the body requires enough insulin.
- Acidosis hyperchloremic: This stems from the loss of sodium bicarbonate. The aim of this is to preserve blood neutrality. Both diarrhea and vomiting can cause this kind of acidosis.
- Lactic acidosis: When the body has too much lactic acid in it, lactic acidosis occurs. The causes may be excessive alcohol use, heart illness, liver damage, seizures, chronic lack of oxygen, low blood sugar, and stroke. Also, a repetitive activity can lead to lactic acid accumulation.
- Renal tubular acidosis: It occurs if the kidneys are unwilling to excrete acids into the urine. Which makes it possible for the blood to become acidic.

Factors of Vulnerability

Factors that may lead to acidosis vulnerability include:

- A high-fat diet and fewer carbohydrate amounts.
- Kidney failure.
- Excess weight.
- Dehydration.
- Poisoning of aspirin or methanol.
- Diabetes.
- Acidosis signs.

Both metabolic and respiratory acidosis share several symptoms. However, the symptoms of acidosis are variable depending on the cause.

Respiratory Acidosis

The following are some of the typical symptoms of respiratory acidosis:

- Drowsiness or exhaustion.
- Rapidly getting tired.
- Confusion.
- Breath difficulty.
- Sleepiness.
- Headaches.

Symptoms of Metabolic Acidosis

The following are some of the typical symptoms of metabolic acidosis:

- Fast and shallow breathing.
- Confusion.
- Tiredness.
- Headaches.
- Sleepiness.
- Absence of hunger.
- Jaundice.
- Elevated heart rate.
- The smelling breath, which can be a symptom of ketoacidosis (diabetic acidosis).

Tests and Diagnosis

If you think you may have acidosis, head to the doctor immediately. Early detection will make a massive difference in your recovery. Physicians can diagnose acidosis using a series of blood tests. An arterial blood gas looks at the concentrations of carbon dioxide and oxygen in the blood. The pH in the blood is revealed as well. The function of the kidney and the balance of the pH is checked by a basic metabolic panel. It also measures the levels of calcium, protein, electrolytes, and blood sugar. When these experiments are done together, they can discern separate types of acidosis. If one is sick with pulmonary acidosis, the specialist may want to examine the state of the lungs. In this, a pulmonary function or a chest x-ray test could be used. If metabolic acidosis is reported, you'd need to give a urine sample. To see how you are correctly extracting acids and bases, doctors will test the pH. Additional tests may be needed to determine the origin of your acidosis.

1.9 WESTERN MEDICINE METHODS FOR CURING ACIDOSIS
Doctors usually need to identify what induces acidosis in order to determine how to treat it. In certain types of acidosis, though, such treatments can be used. E.g., the doctor will give you sodium bicarbonate to boost the pH in the blood. This can be achieved either by intravenous (IV) drip or mouth. Medication can require the treatment of the source of other types of acidosis.

Acidosis in Respiration
Furthermore, procedures for this condition are meant to strengthen the lungs. E.g., you can be given medicines to dilate the airway. You can also be supplied with oxygen or a continuous positive airway pressure (CPAP) device. The CPAP machine can help you breathe whether you have an obstructed airway or muscle exhaustion.

Acidosis in Metabolism

For the various kinds of metabolic acidosis, they each have their own treatments. People with hyperchloremic acidosis should be given oral sodium bicarbonate. Acidosis arising from kidney disease may be treated with sodium citrate. In order to maintain the pH, diabetics with ketoacidosis receive insulin and IV fluids. Treatment of lactic acidosis can include IV fluids, bicarbonate vitamins, antibiotics, oxygen, based on the source.

Problems

Acidosis can contribute to the following health problems without timely treatment:

- Kidney stones.
- Chronic complications with the kidneys.
- Kidney failure.
- Bone illness.
- Delay in growth.

1.10 ACIDOSIS TREATMENT AND PREVENTION THROUGH DR. SEBI'S RECOMMENDED FOODS

You should switch to Dr. Sebi's lifestyle philosophy and diet plan to help prevent and manage metabolic and respiratory acidosis. It will assist you in achieving the following objectives:

- Maintain a healthier weight. because of obesity, you may find it more difficult to breathe properly.
- Acidosis in metabolism.
- Keep hydrated with plenty of water and other fluids.
- Keeping diabetes under control.
- Avoid eating alcohol.

People usually fully heal from acidosis by keeping to Dr. Sebi's diet schedule and approved goods. It can cause complications with respiratory failure, organ function, kidney failure if Dr. Sebi's diet schedule is not applied. Severe acidosis may cause shock or even death.

How well you recover from acidosis depends upon the cause and the capacity to faithfully follow Dr. Sebi's diet plans.

Chapter 2

Dr. Sebi's Philosophy and Health Benefits of the Diet

D r. Sebi was a pathologist, herbalist, biochemist, and naturalist. In North America, Central and South America, Africa, and the Caribbean, he researched and directly experienced herbs and established a special technique and philosophy for treating the human body with herbs deeply embedded in over 30 years of practice. Dr. Sebi, whose given name was Alfredo Bowman, was born in the village of Langa in Spanish Honduras on 26 November 1933. Dr. Sebi was a self-educated guy. "His early days of playing and watching the river and in the trees, along with instruction from his grandmother, provided Sebi the base to be faithful to the reality in his later life. He took signs of being faithful to the procession of life from his beloved grandmother, Mama Hay."

A self-educated man who was afflicted with asthma, diabetes, impotence, and obesity, Sebi moved to the United States. Sebi became an herbalist in Mexico following failed treatments with mainstream physicians and popular western medicine. He started developing natural vegetation cell food compounds tailored to intercellular cleansing and the revitalization of all the cells that make up the human body, achieving tremendous healing results from all his ailments. For 30 years of his life, Dr. Sebi devoted himself to creating a new approach that he could acquire only by years of scientific experience. He started exchanging the compounds with others, which gave rise to Dr. Sebi's cell food, motivated by the personal healing experience and expertise he acquired. Dr. Sebi produced a line of natural vegetable cell food compounds used for intercellular cleansing and cellular revitalization upon discovering the cure he had found by herbs. He developed a theory, and, consequently, the lifestyle of Dr. Sebi that stresses the intake of foods and vitamins that eliminate the mucus-producing disease by achieving an alkaline condition in your body. According to Dr. Sebi, infection in an area of the body is the product of mucus build-up. A build-up of mucus in the lungs, for example, is pneumonia, while diabetes is surplus mucus in the pancreas. The diet comprises a detailed list of plants, fruits, nuts, grains, seeds, herbs, and oils that have been certified. Dr. Sebi's diet is called a vegan diet since animal products are not allowed. Sebi claims you have to obey the diet regularly for the remainder of your life for the body to repair itself.

2.1 DR. SEBI'S PHILOSOPHY

The late Dr. Sebi developed this strictly plant-based diet. The advocates of the theory of Sebi quite reasonably assert that when combined with unique nutrients, it decreases the incidence of disease. Dr. Sebi assumed that the illness was induced by mucus and acidity. He held that the body should be detoxified by consuming some foods while eliminating others, creating an alkaline environment that could decrease the incidence of illness symptoms. Plant-based diets can improve wellness in certain scenarios, and adequate essential nutrients are provided in Dr. Sebi's diet to maintain the body balanced.

The Western approach to illness was thought to be ineffective by Dr. Sebi. He assumed that mucus and acidity induced illness, rather than bacteria and viruses, for instance. A central idea behind the diet is that only in acidic conditions will the disease survive. In order to avoid or eliminate sickness, the purpose of the diet is to achieve an alkaline condition in the body. Botanical medicines that can detoxify the body are given by the diet. Some of these therapies are labeled nutrients of African Bio-Mineral Balance. The diet of Dr. Sebi offers various advantages compared with other diets focused on vegetables. Consuming more whole fruits and vegetables may have beneficial health implications. If it is a target, it could also encourage a person to lose weight. However, the constraints on the diet of Dr. Sebi can be regulated by ensuring that the body consumes adequate nutrients, including vitamin B-12, by supplementation, if appropriate.

Dr. Sebi claimed the infection was triggered by bodily fluid and sharpness. He believed that the body could be detoxified by consuming some items while keeping a strategic gap from others, achieving a soluble speech that could minimize the risk of sickness symptoms. Dr. Sebi's diet will avoid and cure illnesses. In some cases, plant-based dietary regimes will benefit well-being since Dr. Sebi's diet provides adequate main supplements to make the body heal.

2.2 HEALTH BENEFITS OF DR. SEBI'S DIET

A study reveals that the plant-based diet of Dr. Sebi may be safe. Because Dr. Sebi was an herbalist, a plant-based diet is one that relies on only or mainly plant-based items. For both, the well-being of an individual and the world, this form of eating can have advantages. A plant-centered diet is viewed by certain persons as excluding any animal products. A diet based on plants is a diet that includes eating much or just food that comes from plants. The word plant-centered diet is known and used by people in numerous forms. It is perceived by certain people as a vegan lifestyle, which entails avoiding all animal products. For some, a diet focused on plants implies that plant foods are the key emphasis of their diets, such as fruits, vegetables, whole grains, nuts, and legumes, however, they may also ingest beef, seafood, or dairy items. A diet focused on plants often relies on organic foods that are nutritious, rather than refined foods. We would now explain what a diet focused on plants is and its health advantages.

2.3 BENEFITS OF WELLNESS

There are several potential health advantages of eating a plant-focused diet, including:

Weight Management
Data shows that persons who consume diets mainly focused on plants appear to have a lower body mass index (BMI) and lower incidence of obesity, diabetes, and heart disease than people who eat meat. Diets focused on plants are rich in fruit and vegetable fiber, complex carbohydrates, and water content. This will help maintain individuals feeling fuller for longer and maximize the utilization of resources while sleeping. A 2009 survey of more than 60,000 individuals has

shown that vegans, led by lacto-ovo vegetarians (those who consume milk and eggs) and pescatarians (people who eat fish but no other meat), have the lowest overall BMI. Non-vegetarians was the category with the greater average BMI.

A 2015 research concluded that more weight-loss occurred from a vegan diet than other less stringent diets. After six months on a vegan diet, participants lost up to 7.5% of their body weight. A 2018 study showed that a diet focused on plants was beneficial for obesity care. In the report, researchers assigned either a vegan diet or a continuation of their daily diet that included meat to 75 persons that were overweight or had obesity.

Only the vegan category reported a substantial weight reduction of 6.5 kilograms (14.33 pounds) after 4 months. The vegan community focused on plants also shed more fat mass and saw insulin sensitivity changes, while those who ate a daily meat diet did not.

Dr. Sebi's Diet Plan Can Help You Lose Weight

Although the diet of Dr. Sebi is not intended for weight loss, if you adopt it, you can lose weight. The diet prevents consuming a Western diet that is rich in sugar, salt, fat, or calories and filled with ultra-processed foods. It advocates an organic, plant-based diet instead. Those that adopt a plant-based diet appear to have smaller rates of heart disease and obesity compared with the Western diet.

A 12-month survey of 65 individuals showed that those who adopted an unrestricted, low-calorie, plant-based whole-food diet lost substantially more weight than those who did not adopt the diet. Those on a diet lost an estimate of 26 pounds (12 kilograms) at the 6-month point, as compared to 3.5 pounds (1.6 kilograms).

Furthermore, except for almonds, beans, avocados, and oils, most items on this diet are poor in calories. Therefore, even though you consume a significant number of permitted items, it is impossible that these would end in a calorie imbalance and contribute to weight gain.

Nevertheless, very-low-calorie diets will typically not be managed in the long run. If they restore a regular diet, most persons who adopt these diets recover weight.

Appetite Control

A 2016 research among young male participants showed that after consuming a plant-based meal comprising peas and beans, they felt more complete and happier than a meat-containing meal.

Altering the Microbiome

Collectively, the term "microbiome" refers to the microorganisms in the gut. Research in 2019 showed that a plant-based diet could favorably modify the microbiome, contributing to less disease danger. Confirming this would, however, take further study.

Lower Risk of Heart Disease and Other Conditions

A 2017 study found that a diet focused on plants would minimize by 40% the risk of coronary heart disease and by half the risk of developing metabolic syndrome and type 2 diabetes.

The lifestyle of Dr. Sebi enables persons to consume natural foods and eliminates unhealthy foods. A 2017 study showed that reducing refined food consumption can increase the general diet's nutritional content in the United States. Research from the Journal of the American Heart Association in 2019 showed that there was a reduced chance of heart failure among middle-aged people who ate diets rich in nutritious plant foods and low in animal products. Consuming less meat, according to the American Heart Association, will also minimize the risk of:

- Stroke.
- High blood pressure.
- High cholesterol.
- Certain cancers.
- Type 2 diabetes.
- Obesity.

Diabetes Prevention and Treatment

By improving insulin sensitivity and reducing insulin tolerance, plant-based diets may help people avoid or control diabetes. Just 2.9% of those on a vegan diet had type 2 diabetes out of the 60,000 persons surveyed in 2009, relative to 7.6% of those on a non-vegetarian diet. People consuming vegetarian diets, including cheese and eggs, have a smaller chance than meat-eaters with type 2 diabetes.

Researchers have often looked at whether it will help to treat diabetes by eating a plant-based diet. The authors of a 2018 study show that vegetarian and vegan diets can help people with diabetes decrease their demands for insulin, lose weight, and boost other metabolic markers. The researchers proposed that physicians might consider suggesting diets focused on plants to individuals with prediabetes or type 2 diabetes. Although the most advantages were seen by veganism, the researchers claimed that all diets centered on plants can contribute to changes. People who choose to adopt a diet focused on plants should adopt one that they know they will maintain in the long run.

Other Potential Benefits of Dr. Sebi's Diet

Its heavy focus on plant-based ingredients is one advantage of Dr. Sebi's diet. The diet encourages a significant variety of vegetables and fruits that are rich in vitamins, minerals, fiber, and plant compounds to be eaten. Decreased irritation and oxidative pressure, and defense against multiple illnesses, have been linked with diets high in vegetables and berries. Those that consumed 7 servings of fruits and vegetables a day had a 26% and 31% lesser risk of cancer and cardiac disease in a survey of 65,226 individuals. Moreover, most people do not consume enough to generate. In a 2018 survey, 9.3% and 12.2% of individuals met the vegetable and fruit guidelines, respectively. Besides, Dr. Sebi's diet encourages consuming whole grains high in fiber and good fats, like almonds, peas, and plant oils. A reduced incidence of heart failure has been correlated with these diets.

2.4 RULES OF DR. SEBI'S DIET

Dr. Sebi's diet guidelines are rather strict. There are eight key laws for Dr. Sebi's diet that must be observed. They concentrate specifically on the elimination of agricultural products, ultra-processed diets, and the usage of patented supplements. You must obey these main guidelines, according to Dr. Sebi's dietary guide:

- Rule 1: You must only eat foods listed in the nutritional guide.
- Rule 2: Drink 1 gallon (3.8 liters) of water every day.
- Rule 3: Take Dr. Sebi's supplements an hour before medications.
- Rule 4: No animal products are permitted.
- Rule 5: No alcohol is allowed.
- Rule 6: Avoid wheat products and only consume the "natural-growing grains" listed in the guide.
- Rule 7: To stop killing your meal, avoid using a microwave.
- Rule 8: Avoid seedless or canned fruits.

2.5 FOODS TO EAT

Diets that restrict extreme-processed foods are linked with better overall diet quality. The nutrition guide for Dr. Sebi outlines various items that are approved on a diet, includes:

- **Fruits:** Cantaloupe, apples, currants, dates, elderberries, figs, papayas, peaches, berries, soft jelly coconuts, plums, pears, seeded key limes, prickly pears, mangoes, seeded melons, tamarind, and West Indies or Latin soursop.
- **Vegetables:** Bell peppers, avocado, cactus flower, cucumber, chickpeas, dandelion greens, lettuce, kale, mushrooms, olives, okra, sea vegetables, tomatoes, squash (only plum, and cherry), and zucchini.
- **Grains:** Amaranth, fonio, Khorasan wheat, wild rice, rye, spelled, quinoa, and teff.
- **Nuts:** Raw sesame seeds, hemp seeds, walnuts raw, Brazil nuts, and tahini butter.
- **Oils:** Coconut oil (raw), avocado oil, grape seed oil, olive oil (raw), sesame oil, and hempseed oil.
- **Herbal teas:** Chamomile, elderberry, fennel, burdock, tila, raspberry, and ginger.
- **Spices:** Basil, cloves, oregano, bay leaf, sweet basil, dill, cayenne, habanero,

achiote, tarragon, sea salt, sage, thyme, pure agave syrup, onion powder, date sugar, powdered and granulated seaweed.

In addition to tea, you can have water. Plus, the allowed grains can be consumed in the shape of pasta, bread, cereal, or wheat. Every product that is leavened with baking powder or yeast is, therefore, forbidden. This diet has a rather strict set of items that are tolerated. It is important to avoid foods that are not included in this chart.

2.6 FOODS TO AVOID

Any food not mentioned in the nutrition guide for Dr. Sebi is not authorized, such as:

- Seedless fruit.
- Eggs.
- Canned vegetables or fruit.
- Dairy.
- Fish.
- Soy products.
- Poultry.
- Processed food, which includes take-out or cafe food.
- Red meat.
- Wheat.
- Fortified foods.
- Sugar (in addition to agave syrup and date sugar).
- Yeast or food rose with yeast.
- Alcohol.
- Food produced with baking powder.

In addition, the diet bans certain herbs, fruits, wheat, nuts, or seeds. The foods mentioned in the manual can only be consumed. Any food which is refined, animal-based, or produced with leavening agents is restricted by the diet. Not approved are some herbs, fruits, beans, nuts, or seeds.

Chapter 3

Mucus, Inflammation, and Dr. Sebi's Curing Methods

Mucus, formed by several lining tissues in the body, is a natural, greasy, and stringy fluid substance. Body function must keep critical organs from drying and provides a defensive and moisturizing sheet. For irritants like pollen, smoke, or bacteria, mucus often serves as a trap. To aid fend off pathogens, it includes bacteria-killing enzymes and antibodies.

A lot of mucus is formed by the body—around 1–1.5 liters every day. Until its development is improved or the consistency of mucus has modified, as may happen with numerous diseases and conditions, we do not appear to see mucus at all.

3.1 COUGHING UP MUCUS

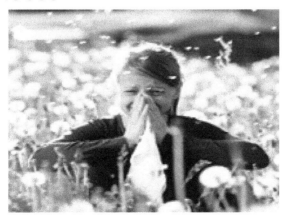

Usually, coughing is a quick evacuation of oxygen from the lungs to clean up the lung airways of:

- Mucus.

- Fluids.
- Acute (less than 3 weeks) or persistent (more than 3 weeks) may be classified as a cough.

3.2 REASONS FOR THE INCREASE IN MUCUS PRODUCTION

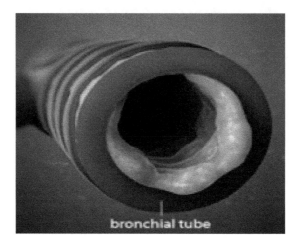
bronchial tube

Popular sources of elevated development of mucus and throwing up mucus are respiratory illnesses such as colds, measles, and sinusitis. Another explanation of why mucus development will rise is due to allergic reactions. In the nasal passages, even the ingestion of spicy foods will spark excess development of mucus.

You may find thickened mucus that may look thicker than average when you are sick with a respiratory infection. It is tougher to flush out this thickened mucus than normal mucus. Many of the hallmark manifestations of the flu or cold are correlated with this mucus. When you are sick, the mucus can look green-yellow as well.

3.3 WHICH AREAS CREATE MUCUS IN THE BODY?

In several places in the body, mucus is formed by mucus glands in the coating of several organ tissues, including:
- Sinuses.
- Mouth.
- Lungs.
- Gastrointestinal tract.
- Throat.
- Nose.

3.4 DIFFERENCE BETWEEN PHLEGM AND MUCUS

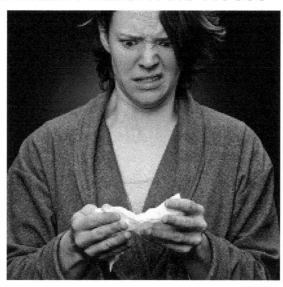

Phlegm is the word used, particularly when excess mucus is formed and coughed up, to describe mucus generated by the respiratory system. The mucus includes the bacteria or viruses accountable for the infection and the infection-fighting body immune system cells (white blood cells) throughout an infection.

Phlegm itself isn't harmful, although it does block the airways when found in significant quantities. Coughing is normally expelled by phlegm, although conditions such as respiratory irritation, sore throat, and runny nose generally follow this.

3.5 WHAT DO DISTINCT COLORS OF PHLEGM AND MUCUS MEAN?

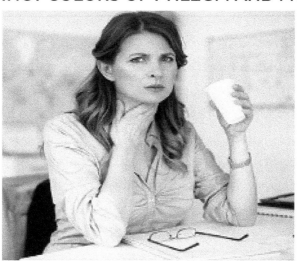

Compared to the usual, transparent, thin mucus, the thickened mucus which surrounds several diseases is frequently thicker and yellow-colored.

Greenish mucus indicates that the mucus includes white blood cells that battle infection.

In upper respiratory infections, brownish or blood-tinged mucus is often widespread, especially if the inside of the nose has been swollen or scratched. Although a small amount of blood in the mucus is common, if there is severe bleeding, you can see a health care provider.

3.6 WHEN IS EXTREME MUCUS AN ISSUE?

Generally, excessive mucus, particularly when covering sinuses or inducing coughing fits, is unpleasant and a nuisance. Thickened mucus and the development of excess mucus cause several undesirable symptoms that include:

- Nasal congestion.
- Runny nose.
- Sinus headache.
- Sore throat.
- Cough.

3.7 UNDERSTANDING CHRONIC INFLAMMATION

Inflammation relates to the mechanism of your body, defending against factors that damage it in an effort to cure itself, such as diseases, fractures, and contaminants. Your body produces chemicals that cause a reaction from your immune system when anything damages your cells.

The release of antibodies and proteins, as well as improved blood flow to the affected region, are involved in this reaction. In the case of acute inflammation, the entire thing normally continues for a few hours or days.

As this reaction lingers, persistent inflammation occurs, keeping the body in a perpetual warning condition. Chronic inflammation may have a detrimental effect on the tissues and organs over time. Some researches indicate that, in a variety of diseases, from cancer to asthma, persistent inflammation may also play a part.

Symptoms of Chronic Inflammation

Acute inflammation, including discomfort, redness, or swelling, frequently produces visible signs. Symptoms of systemic inflammation that are typical include:

- Fatigue.
- Fever.
- Mouth sores.
- Rashes.
- Abdominal pain.
- Chest pain.

These symptoms can range from mild to severe, and last for several months or years.

Causes of Chronic Inflammation

Chronic inflammation may be caused by many factors, including:

- Untreated sources, such as an illness or fracture, of acute inflammation.
- An inflammatory disease causing a misplaced attack on healthy tissue by the immune system.
- Long-time exposure to irritants, such as toxic contaminants or dirty air.

Bear in mind that not everyone induces systemic inflammation. Additionally, there is no apparent causal explanation for certain forms of systemic inflammation.

Experts also agree that persistent inflammation can also lead to several causes, such as:

- Smoking.
- Obesity.
- Alcohol.
- Chronic stress.

The Negative Impact of Chronic Inflammation on the Body

The inflammatory reaction of your body will ultimately start destroying healthy cells, tissues, and organs when you have persistent inflammation. This can lead to DNA damage, tissue death, and internal scarring over time.

Many of these are correlated with the emergence of several diseases, including:

- Heart disease.
- Cancer.
- Rheumatoid arthritis.
- Asthma.
- Obesity.

3.8 HOW IS CHRONIC INFLAMMATION TREATED THROUGH CHANGES IN DIET

A normal aspect of the healing phase is inflammation. But as it becomes persistent, to decrease the chance of long-term injury, it is necessary to get it under control. In controlling chronic inflammation, what you consume will play both a positive and a negative function.

Foods to Eat

There are anti-inflammatory properties in several foods. This involves foods which are rich in antioxidants and polyphenols, such as:

- Leafy greens, like spinach and kale.
- Olive oil.
- Tomatoes.
- Nuts.
- Fatty fish, like sardines, salmon, and mackerel.
- Fruits, like blueberries, cherries, and oranges.

You should suggest trying Dr. Sebi's diet if you want to reconsider your eating patterns. An analysis showed that there were lower markers of inflammation in participants observing this diet.

Foods to Avoid

The following foods can increase inflammation in some people:

- Refined carbohydrates, such as white bread and pastries.
- Fried foods, such as French fries.

- Red meat.
- Processed meat, such as hot dogs and sausage.

Try to limit the consumption of these things if you're looking to reduce inflammation. You don't need to remove them entirely; just aim to consume them just periodically. Your chance of many severe ailments is raised by systemic inflammation. Using blood samples, the doctor will detect inflammation. You will help reduce the chance of inflammation by taking drugs, vitamins, and consuming an anti-inflammation diet. As well as lowering the stress levels, avoiding smoke and alcohol, and keeping a healthy body weight will both help to reduce your risk.

3.9 DR. SEBI'S PHILOSOPHY ON TREATING AND CURING MUCOUS AND INFLAMMATION

Dr. Sebi did not identify or recommend pharmaceuticals for the condition. He appeared to be a culinary expert and made nutrition-related proposals. At least one hour before starting your medicine, it is advised that you take the products so that the nutrients given will be completely assimilated.

Products from Dr. Sebi are labeled as food for natural vegetation cells. As a consequence, you would have nourished your cells before you take them and will not have much of an appetite.

The treatment investigates and describes the origins of the illness, not just the signs. Dr. Sebi also claimed that the origin of the sickness was mucus. The disease will occur in the body where mucus has been collected, according to the philosophy of Dr. Sebi. Since the food compounds of the natural vegetation cells are engineered to remove mucus from a given region of the body, it is often important to clean the body as a whole. The special and exclusive features of the compounds of Dr. Sebi are the way they function to cleanse and nourish the whole body.

You will successfully reverse pathologies through this method. As the herbs used have a natural origin, the substances begin to unleash their cleansing properties 14 days after they are first taken. Adhering to the dietary recommendations is an equally significant part of Dr. Sebi's diet policy. In combination with dietary improvements, Dr. Sebi's herbal compounds function to give the body the right climate to maintain optimum wellness. It also aims to achieve the most positive effects for your well-being by consuming a gallon of natural spring water every day.

Chapter 4

Alkaline Diet and Its Advantages

D r. Sebi's African approach to illness relies on natural botanical remedies to detoxify and cleanse the body, returning it to a more alkaline state from the acidity that causes illness and disease. An integral aspect of the transition is natural food compounds from vegetable cells. By removing stored toxins and replacing depleted minerals, cellular foods can rejuvenate degraded cell tissue, especially those consumed by acidity.

The primary organs impacted include the head, stomach, gall bladder, kidneys, lymph glands, and colon. Cell foods are an important part of a healing and a person's dietary ecosystem, with inclusive therapeutic programs centered on healing and around the whole individual and their diet and well-being.

Dr. Sebi's program does not prescribe or distribute medicines for diseases. Essentially, the program provides nutritional consulting and creates suggestions relevant to eating. In this way, none of the information given here is supposed to accompany any program prescribed by the doctor for you, nor does it conflict with any medication that you are taking. It is recommended that you take the products at least an hour before taking the medication so that the nutrients supplied can be thoroughly assimilated.

4.1 WHAT IS ALKALINE DIET?

The Alkaline diet is based on the idea that replacing acid-forming ingredients with alkaline foods will improve your well-being. Alkaline nutrition can help battle diseases such as cancer that are serious. It will improve well-being by restricting junk food and embracing more plant foods. The Alkaline diet is often referred to as the Acid-Alkaline diet. The idea is that the food can influence the measurement of the body's pH value, alkalinity, or acidity. Your metabolism is also related to the transfer of power from food. In each, a chemical reaction is required that breaks down a tough mass. However, the chemical reactions in the body happen in a slow and controlled way. Similarly, the things you consume leave an "ash" residue known as metabolic waste. This metabolic waste is likely to be acidic, alkaline, or neutral. Metabolic waste will directly affect the body's acidity. In other words, whenever you eat anything that leaves acidic waste, it renders the blood more acidic. When you eat anything that leaves alkaline waste, it renders the blood more alkaline. According to the acid-ash hypothesis, acidic ash is thought to make you susceptible to illness and disease, while alkaline ash is considered protective. By consuming more alkaline ingredients, you must be able to "alkalize" the body and improve your health. Food components that produce acidic ash include sulfur, meat, and phosphorus, while alkaline components include potassium, calcium, and magnesium.

The Alkaline diet is similar to any diet that you've heard in the manner that it will prevent, reverse, and even stop some infections and cancers. In the pharmaceutical and herbal fields, it has been demonstrated to be fact. For instance, cancer patients who'd been put on an Alkaline diet were able to increase their pH levels, allowing cancer cells to become ineffective (at 7.4 pH) and ultimately die (at 7.8 pH). Any other disease is the same concern, such as asthma, STDs, and arthritis, even the big one, AIDS. The concept of eating a healthy Acid-Alkaline diet is a difficult one because if you inspire the body to become even mildly acidic, you risk:

- Incapability to breathe oxygen, which causes the individual to slowly suffocate.
- Free radical damage increases and leads to cancerous mutations in the blood.
- Premature aging (a significant sign predictor of the body's nutrient/

oxygen shortfall).
- Coronary system injury due to blood vessel restrictions, inadequate oxygen in the tissue, and hypertension.
- Obesity leads to diabetes.
- Stones in the bladder and kidney.
- Slower healing of wounds and illness.
- An immune system deficit.
- Higher control thresholds, persistent weakness, and depression.
- Weak, brittle bones that may lead to osteoporosis, bone, and hip fractures.
- Pressure attributable to lactic acid accumulation in the tissues and knees.
- In the body, it is simpler for illnesses and disorders to develop.
- Ketoacidosis, liver/kidney progressive diseases, severe diarrhea, and adrenal gland insufficiency.

This information is troubling for a lot of people. Once again, there are facts to back it up. However, you have to look for it, and the pharmaceutical company won't place this in front of you.

4.2 WHAT YOU CAN AND CAN'T EAT

Some berries, fruits, tofu, soybean, certain rice, nuts, and legumes are alkaline-promoting plants, so they're perfectly acceptable. Dairy, meat, most fruits, and processed items like milk, frozen, and packaged food, go on the acid side, and are not allowed, such as fast foods and popcorn. Often, traditional Alkaline diets reduce the use of alcohol or caffeine. Certain food classes believe themselves to be neutral, alkaline, or acidic:
- Acidic: poultry, meat, fish, eggs, alcohol, dairy, and grains.
- Alkaline: nuts, vegetables, legumes, and fruits.
- Neutral: starches, sugars, and natural fats.

The metabolic waste remaining from the processing of foods can also affect the alkalinity or acidity of the body directly. The Alkaline diet includes typical products with a pH ranking of 7 or higher (meaning non-starch and non-hybrid). It uses a mixture of vegetables, berries, nuts, rice, herbs, and seeds. Acidic ingredients such as coffee/caffeine, meat, butter, rice, potato starches, sugar, wheat, and eggs are often removed. It is a healthy vegan diet because soy, potatoes, and rice are eaten by many vegans. All plant-based diets are not alkaline, and old farmers and the scientists who promote a balanced Acid-Alkaline diet have conjugated many of them today. Remember, it is crucial. And you will find that they still support their goods over all others. What were the nutritious foods in high school that they told you to consume?

The list goes on, like broccoli, apples, whole wheat, bananas, celery, spinach, rice, cauliflower, pineapples, oranges, peanut butter, kidney beans, massive tomatoes. You can get natural (heaven-made) items, such as turnips, peaches, pears, plums, walnuts, olives, etc.; the oranges, strawberries, onions, and bananas, are not bad. However, it comes down to selecting the good one for eating. Carrots, pineapples, and celery are made up of two different classes and did not exist until the beginning of time.

You will determine whether a product is a mixture by measuring the pH level and if it contains starch. Carrots, corn, and peas, etc., are producing starch and being acidic. Starch doesn't normally exist in nature. It is a chemical that forms as a hybrid; the starch is the glue that allows the two to combine. You will see individuals treat diseases with alkaline and acidic ingredients (incorporating leafy greens, lettuce, peppers, apples, and more), but since it is paired with alkaline-rich ones, it simply balances out as an Alkaline diet. Then why not exclude acidic goods entirely? It is necessary to know the African diet if you are of African descent, as they say, that blueberries are acidic, which is true for Caucasians, but in our bodies, it is extremely alkalizing. The newest invention that takes the body to a completely new degree of unhealthy level with onions, rice, soy, and a few other things we consume every day is genetically engineered goods. So, watch out for seedless fruits.

4.3 REGULAR PH LEVELS IN YOUR BODY

When taking into consideration the Alkaline diet, it is important to remember pH. Put simply: pH is an indicator of how alkaline or acidic anything is.

The pH value goes from 0 to 14:

- **Acidic:** 0.0 to 6.9.
- **Alkaline (or basic):** 7.1 to 14.0.
- **Neutral:** 7.0.

Several supporters of this diet propose that individuals monitor the pH of the urine in order to ensure that it is not acidic (below 7) and is alkaline (over 7). It's necessary to note, however, that pH varies greatly within the body. While certain parts are acidic, others are alkaline, and there is no degree fixed. The stomach is packed with hydrochloric acid, which renders the pH of 2-3.5 highly acidic. This acidity is important for breaking down food. On the other hand, human blood, with a pH of 7.36-7.44, is mostly slightly alkaline. As the blood pH falls out of the normal range, it can be fatal if left uncontrolled. This occurs during other illness cycles, such as ketoacidosis caused by insulin, excessive alcohol, and starvation. The pH value checks a material's alkalinity or acidity. For starters, stomach acid is highly acidic, while blood is slightly alkaline.

4.4 FOOD AFFECTS THE PH LEVELS WITHIN YOUR BODY

The blood pH must stay stable for health. If it were to dip below the normal range, the cells would quit working, and you would die very quickly if untreated. For this reason, the body has many effective ways of closely regulating its pH equilibrium. This is called acid-base homeostasis.

In fact, food can influence the pH of the blood in people. Similarly, the diet will change the pH content of the urine also. The excretion of acids in the urine is one of the main factors the body regulates blood pH. Many hours afterward, when you eat a massive steak, the urine can become more acidic as the body clears the metabolic waste from the bloodstream.

The amounts of blood pH are strictly regulated by the body. In healthy people, diet significantly affects blood pH, which can modify urinary pH.

4.5 THE PROMISE OF ALKALINE DIETS

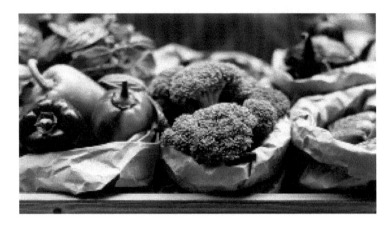

For the Alkaline diet or the Acid-Alkaline diet, you can reduce weight and stop risks such as inflammation and cancer. The theory is that such products, like refined sugar, meat, wheat, and packaged foods, cause the body to produce acid that is harmful to you. Thus, according to the "research" behind this scheme, eating particular foods that make the body more alkaline can protect against such ailments as well as shed pounds.

This diet should predominantly be entirely vegetarian. That also works with vegans, in that milk is off-limits. The diet excludes wheat, but in order to fully remove gluten, you will need to review food labels carefully since gluten is not present in wheat. In addition to wheat, the diet nullifies many of the other main triggers of food allergies, including milk, beef, peanuts, seafood, walnuts, and shellfish. For people who try to avoid fat and sugar is also perfect.

4.6 HEALTH BENEFITS OF ALKALINE DIETS

For a large variety of chronic illnesses and symptoms, including the daily development of mucus and cold headaches, anxiety, women's disorders, such as polycystic ovarian cysts and ovaries, and low energy in general, this alternative Alkaline diet works wonders. It has led to substantial weight-loss among those who have pursued it and makes common sense because of the large number of vegetables and fruits and the scarcity of processed food in the diet. An Alkaline diet is not prescribed for infants, persons with heart failure, kidney injury; or pregnant or breastfeeding women should first consult their doctor.

On this Alkaline diet, the foods that people consume will help to maintain stable body weight. Using this will help avoid health conditions that are connected to excess weight, including diabetes. Research indicates that an Alkaline diet will improve well-being. Alkaline diets minimize a person's consumption of processed and fatty meats and allow people to consume more fresh fruits and vegetables. It has many health benefits. Some of the benefits offered to people by Alkaline diets are described in the next topics.

4.7 CURES STDS AND HERPES

STDs to be called venereal diseases or VD. They are one of the most dangerous and contagious diseases. More than 65 million people suffer from incurable STDs. There are 19.9 million new cases identified annually; many of these diseases develop in persons between 15-24 years of age and can have long-term consequences. STDs are extreme disorders that require treatment. These STDs, like HIV, if not be treated, and can be lethal. Through learning more about STDs, you will learn how to protect yourself. An STD can harm your vaginal, anal, or oral route. Trichomonas can also be induced by interaction with moist or dirty objects such as blankets, wet clothing, or toilet seats, although a sexual disease is more frequently transmitted. You are at high risk if:

- Having more than one intimate partner.
- Having sex with someone who had many mates.
- Not using a condom while having sex.
- Sharing needles while delivering intravenous drugs.
- Swapping sex for drugs.

You do not realize you have those STDs until your reproductive organs (make you infertile), heart, vision, or other organs are damaged; an STD can compromise the immune system, making one more prone to other infections. Pelvic Inflammatory Disorder (PID) is a complication of chlamydia and gonorrhea that can render women unable to bear babies. It could get you killed as well. If you transfer an STD to a newborn baby, the child can suffer permanent harm or death.

What Causes STDs?

In STDs, just about every form of the disease is involved. Bacterial STDs contain gonorrhea, syphilis, and chlamydia. Viral STDs include HIV, hepatitis B, vaginal herpes, and genital warts. Trichomonas is caused by a parasite. The germs which trigger STDs hide in hair, semen, even in saliva and vaginal secretions. Some species are transmitted by anal, oral, and vaginal sex. While some, like those that cause genital warts and genital herpes, may be transferred by skin contact. Through sharing personal items, such as razors, toothbrushes, you can get hepatitis B from someone who has it.

Get Your STDs and Other Chronic Conditions Cured by the Alkaline Diet Plan

You can spend hours just making a list of the multiple diet programs sponsored by various clinicians, diet plan agencies, and alternative therapies. There is one diet, though, which is not only very popular but is heavily focused on science, though traditional and alternative medicine experts disagree slightly about whether it's good for you.

Herpes, HIV, STDs, hepatitis, and genital warts are persistent conditions that can be managed by using Dr. Sebi's Alkaline diet protocol. It mainly consists of fresh produce, various seeds, and nuts as well (green vegetables). Hepatitis B can become chronic, but it is often possible to control it. In the body, there are different pH ranges; for example, the liver is very acidic so that it can break down food, whereas the blood is moderately alkaline, just below 7.5 for most individuals.

The theory behind the Alkaline diet is that not only does maintain the body's pH levels aid with weight management. It also tends to reduce common diseases, cancers, and other serious diseases. Followers of the Alkaline diet looked at history in order to develop this theory. Long ago, individuals ate food that was normal, not processed, from plants and animals. New foods have been used in the human diet over time and have become classics of it. Salt, refined grains, sugar, animal products, and processed meat (were once domesticated) were included. All of these foods are acidic in nature. They produce acid when digested while natural foods are mainly alkaline.

The theory centers mainly on the notion that every diet high in acidic foods upsets the body's natural pH equilibrium, implying that vital minerals such as potassium, magnesium, and calcium are lost as the body tries to maintain or regain its pH balance. The imbalance also leads to bone deterioration, leaving people more prone to bone disorder, with weight-gain, sickness, and serious diseases such as cancer and heart disease. In reality, in an acidic setting, cancer is known to grow, so the extent of body pH is an important cause of why cancer is far more widespread than it used to be.

An Alkaline diet primarily includes foods that are natural and partly alkaline in order to keep the pH levels of the body healthy and right. The complementary medicine group considers an Alkaline diet to be of substantial benefit for the following variables. In traditional medicine, many people believe that the body's pH level cannot be chemically "manipulated" and that cancer inevitably creates the acidic environment in which it grows. All nutritionists agree that a diet high in alkaline foods such as nuts, vegetables, and bananas (with water) is very good for someone, in general, and that consuming a lot of acidic foods such as processed, carbohydrates, and animal protein is bad. Almost all vegetables, legumes, and grains, some seeds and nuts (but no cashews, walnuts, and almonds) are used in a large portion of this diet. Some foods are encouraged; others are only to be eaten in moderation. Most fresh fruits are contained in this group, and others are strictly forbidden.

4.8 ACIDITY CAUSES CANCER, BUT YOU CAN PROTECT YOURSELF BY STICKING TO RECOMMENDED ALKALINE DIETS

Cancer often spreads in an acidic environment and can be treated or even healed by an Alkaline diet. Tumors grow better in acidic environments. The analysis proposes a connection between cancer and an acid-forming diet. Alkaline nutrition has the ability to heal tumors and facilitate chemotherapy. Significant results from a 2010 survey suggest that by reducing meat consumption and eating more fruits, herbs, and whole grains, cancer may be prevented. The study looked at data from the Prospective Review of European Cancer and Diet from 2010. It was reported that by consuming vitamin A, vitamin C, fiber, and a plant-based diet, cancer risk could be minimized. The American Cancer Society (ACS) recommends a diet that is equal to an Alkaline diet. The ACS advises that it is possible to stop cooked meats, soft drinks, and some high-fat ingredients;

instead, it is more beneficial to consume a diet rich in fruits, whole grains, and vegetables.

4.9 PROMOTING WEIGHT-LOSS

Often strategies can help people lose weight. In the end, losing weight depends on consuming fewer calories than one is burning. Lower fat and calorie diets can support weight-loss, but only if an individual is physically involved and eats a healthy and varied diet. It seems that an Alkaline diet is limited in calories, helping people lose weight. Overweight is an issue of acidity. Besides living an 80/20 Alkaline diet, there are two weight-holding techniques. First, one can introduce healthier alkaline fats into their diet; this is such that, when one eats fat, they will lose calories. Preferably, 50 to 70% of the regular diet can comprise of fats like coconut oil, avocados, natural seeds, and nuts such as hemp, chia, and almonds whole nut butter (not peanut butter) like cacao, almonds, coconut, and also nutritious Omega-3 fish like wild-caught salmon. The second technique is to try something called occasionally fasting. For this, you ought to eat 3 alkaline meals per day and discourage feeding in between. And you want to eat these 3 meals (for say, 9-5) in 8 hours. In the off-hours, you can stay well hydrated with herbal teas, lemon water, and green juices. By doing so, you lower your insulin levels, and the body moves from a glucose burning as its primary fuel to fat-burning as its supply.

4.10 TREATING OR PREVENTING HEART DISEASE

Cardiac disease is the major cause of death in the U.S. lifestyle indicators, including poor nutrition and inadequate amounts of exercise, are essential considerations. An Alkaline diet can normally raise levels of growth hormones. The research indicates that growth hormone improves the composition of the body and lowers risk factors for heart disease. Alkaline diets also seem low in sugar and cholesterol, naturally supporting healthy body weight and reducing risk factors for cardiovascular disease. Red and dried meats are frequently diminished or eliminated, removing a large contributor to dietary heart disease.

4.11 IMPROVING LEVELS OF GROWTH HORMONES

Improved cardiac safety is only one potential advantage of reaching elevated growth hormone levels. Improving levels of growth hormones, especially cognition and memory, may also promote improved functioning of the brain. There is some evidence that the overall quality of life is increased by growth hormones. Good data are available that link an Alkaline diet to increases in growth hormone levels. Every study has shown that the adjustment of a strongly acidic environment with some supplements such as bicarbonate can promote alkalinity.

4.12 IMPROVING BACK PAIN

A significant body of research suggests that substituting the diet with alkaline elements reduces the effects of back pain. In this research, the benefits of an Alkaline diet were assessed, so Alkaline diets aid with chronic pain.

4.13 PROMOTING HEALTHY MUSCLES

People tend to lose muscle mass when they age. In a human, this increases the risk of falls and fractures, and it may also contribute to exhaustion and chronic pain. A 2013 study gives preliminary confirmation that an Alkaline diet may boost muscle fitness. Researchers examined 2,689 females in a long-term twin study. They found a small but significant improvement in muscle mass among females adopting a more Alkaline diet.

4.14 ALKALINE DIET HELPS TREAT DIABETIC PEOPLE

Alkaline diets must maintain the alkaline food is 70-80% of the food consumed. This stimulates food from the acidic culture to be eaten, albeit in limited quantities. You can question whether such products, including berries, are included in the group of alkaline foods. The hypothesis is that, after digestion, the materials have an alkaline influence. The Alkaline diet tends to protect the body from becoming more acidic than it needs to be, thus keeping the body from having to take the same number of corrective measures to preserve the body's usual pH level. In the Alkaline diet, there is a clear focus on plants, and the restriction of grains is like the restrictions on low-carb diets. The grains which can be used have a comparatively less glycemic load compared with other grains. It doesn't have to be a vegetarian diet because acidic items can be up to

30% of the food intake. For a vegetarian diet, the transition to an Alkaline diet may be easier than for those who are not vegetarian. The degree of flexibility offered by the diet means that the diet can be conveniently customized to avoid any food shortages.

Diabetes and Mind-Boggling Facts About Diabetes

Here are some of the amazing statistics:

- $1 in each $5 in health care cost to help patients with diabetes.
- Across America, 8.1 million people are projected to be living with undiagnosed diabetes.
- Diabetes affects one in four Americans over the age of 65.

Until we learn how an Alkaline diet could theoretically cure diabetes, let us first speak about the fundamentals and bases of diabetes. There are two forms of diabetes, type 1 diabetes and type 2 diabetes, overall. Just type 2 diabetes is addressed here. This is the type that usually occurs later in life and maybe handled by dietary changes as well. For type 2 diabetes, certain products in the body through not work optimally. Second, the body may not generate enough of the insulin hormone that is needed to pass glucose (sugar) from the blood to the cells to supply energy. Conversely, with type 2 diabetes, the body may still produce adequate insulin, although this hormone does not act properly. We usually refer to this as "insulin tolerance," which may lead to excessive blood sugar levels and diabetes as a consequence.

Causes of Diabetes

First of all, researchers understand that there is a hereditary component of diabetes. Any people develop diabetes because of their DNA, rather than the complications of their diet and lifestyle. Consequently, meat, exercise habits, and movement will play a role in diabetes as well. Most of us have encountered the popular recommendations for a healthy weight, exercising our body regularly, and avoiding sugary, fried items. But what if there was a special aspect at risk here? Studies suggest that an acidic diet also has a part in causing diabetes. The theory is that thanks to such foods, our blood pH reduces and turns more acidic. This is said to lead to illnesses of all sorts. On the other hand, it is assumed that it will heal and prevent illness by eating the foods that alkalize the blood. In many large-scale trials, a strong and compelling link was discovered between an Alkaline diet and increased insulin resistance. It has also been shown that the incidence of having diabetes is decreased by this advantage.

How Do We Achieve Better Results for Diabetes With the Alkaline Diet?

To explain why diabetes can be improved by alkalizing diets, there's a need to understand how the bodies absorb acid and alkaline foods. Our bodies create a lot of mineral chemicals and cations that are normal digestion by-products as one eats food (such as potassium, phosphorus, calcium, and magnesium). However, these by-products tend to be differentiated from "acid" and "alkaline" foods and have a different influence on pH.

Acidic Foods

- The synthesis of more sulfate during the metabolic stage.
- Increase the dietary acid load.

Alkaline Foods

- A tendency to have a higher protein/low in potassium content.
- The by-products metabolically of eating these foods are buffered by hydrogen ions that reduce acidity.

Decreases the Fatty Acid Load

It is extremely important to note here that the body performs an excellent job at maintaining the pH levels via kidneys as well as the respiratory system. The blood pH is strictly regulated in healthy people, between 7.35 and 7.45. When we are outside this set, we become seriously sick. On the bottom end of the normal pH scale, quite acidic, a reliably high dietary acid load would also sustain the body. And scientists agree that what improves the risk of diabetes is, to minimize insulin exposure, a drop in blood pH—even within the "healthy" range. On the other hand, alkalizing the blood was shown to improve insulin resistance and the ability of the cells to metabolize glucose.

One popular theory is that a very mild process of acidosis could impair the ability of insulin to bind to cells. Another theory is that large loads of dietary acid will cause the liver to develop and release more glucose—something that is expected to occur only when the body wants more energy during meals, and exercise or sleep. The irony remains that many large-scale experiments reveal a strong link between the more alkaline eating behaviors and stronger blood glucose and insulin control. This is because most alkaline foods, based around vegetables, are content that we would all eat more of anyway. Eating more of such alkalizing plants gives far greater benefits than the opportunity to prevent diabetes, with few Americans satisfying their usual criteria for fruits and vegetables. In the same manner, most "acidic products"—including red and dry meats, hard cheese, starch, processed/fried foods, and beer—can be eaten in abundance (or not at all) for other health reasons, in addition to the lowered risk of diabetes. So, if you're diabetic or not, eat some fruits and vegetables that are alkalizing, and they're guaranteed to like you again. Often, it's good to remember the analysis informs us why, too.

Tips for Diabetic People

Diet management is important for diabetics. In addition to assisting with weight-reduction and controlling blood sugar levels, it also ensures the proper acid-alkaline ratio. The food we eat affects the pH level of the body; eating certain foods can increase the level of acid, while others will reduce it. It is important to maintain the acid content under check, and one easy way to do it is to eat alkaline foods. The acid-alkaline balance needs to be controlled when one is a diabetic person. Kidney problems in people suffering from diabetes are common. In this way, the kidneys extract waste from the body and detoxify the blood. Extra acid and glucose in the blood destroy the kidneys, which then begin to worsen and avoid working for some time. High acid levels in the body may lead to diabetic ketoacidosis (DKA), where acids accumulate in the urine and blood. If not treated, it can be life-threatening.

The Alkaline diet stresses the intake of fresh items and fewer quantities of carbohydrates and dairy, which will boost the acid content by one second. It is one means of ensuring that healthy food is eaten and thereby prevents the stomach from acid attacks. Consuming rich alkaline foods often allows the body to be detoxified, and the pH level of the body to be preserved.

Avoid Eating Refined Foods

Refined means without flesh in general. Even if it brushes the peas and grains you eat and modifies them, don't consume them. There's a reason why certain foods have meat in the first place. Many refined food items very quickly burn sugar since it has low-fiber material. The same also happens to processed goods, and this would raise the amounts of acid

First thing every morning, stop acidic foods or beverages.

If you have the habit of drinking tea or coffee, refrain. These beverages are acidic in nature, restricting the metabolism of carbohydrates and vitamins from becoming ingested in the morning. It enhances stress hormones that lead to insulin resistance. These fundamental yet effective diet tips can go a long way towards helping us maintain the acid-alkaline balance.

4.15 LUPUS AND ALKALINE DIET

Lupus is a chronic inflammatory condition in which your body's immune system becomes hyperactive and damages the tissue that is healthy and normal. The symptoms are pain, swelling, and damage to tissues, skin, kidneys, heart, oxygen, and lungs. Because of its diverse nature, people sometimes refer to lupus as the disease of 1,000 faces. People in the United States report approximately 16,000 new cases of lupus each year, as per the Lupus Foundation of America, and up to 1.5 million people could be diagnosed with the condition. The Foundation notes that lupus impacts women in particular, and it is most likely to develop between the ages of 15 to 44. Lupus is not a viral disease. An individual is unwilling to pass it physically or in some other manner to another person. Women with lupus may, however, give birth to children who, in exceptional instances, acquire a form of lupus. There is neonatal lupus as well. Various causes of lupus exist. It quickly addresses only Systemic Lupus Erythematosus (SLE), while other forms include neonatal lupus, discoid, and drug-induced.

Systemic Lupus Erythematosus

SLE is the most common type of lupus. It is a disorder that is systemic. This indicates that it has an impact on the body. The symptoms may range between mild and extreme.

It is more severe than other types of lupus, such as discoid lupus, because it can impair any of your body's organs or organ systems. Inflammation may be induced and affects the skin, lungs, liver, limbs, blood, heart, or a combination of these. Usually, this disorder passes into phases. There will be no symptoms in the person at times of remission. Just before a flare-up, the condition is present, and symptoms occur.

Lupus Treatment With an Alkaline Diet

Several diet groups will boost the effects of lupus. There are many widely known causes that, aside from multiple substances that may contribute to symptoms, can trigger lupus to flare up. Because of this, identifying which foods relate to feeling great or worse can be quite complicated. Alfalfa has been reported to lower muscle pain and general fatigue, and garlic strengthens the immune system. Of course, everyone should forbid saturated fats and trans fats, but this is something everyone knows. And, given the possibility of heart disease among lupus sufferers, it is recommended to minimize red meat in favor of a diet that contains more fish. Eventually, since more of the medications for lupus patients to be used to treat their disease will produce a reduction in calcium-rich foods, bone density should be part of the regular diet. These include milk, broccoli, spinach, cheese, yogurt, tofu, beans, and dark-leafy vegetables that are low-fat. Salt increases blood pressure and may boost the risk of heart failure in people with lupus, so it should be minimized or eliminated as quickly as possible. Remember that some alkaline alternatives include spices, such as cloves, curry, turmeric, ginger, and other seasonings. The single largest source of assistance in creating a lifestyle that will help you handle lupus flare-ups relies on the adherence to an Alkaline diet routine. With increased food intake helpful in keeping an alkaline balance, it will find it simpler to conduct the functions of the liver, such as the kidney and heart. The goal is to track impacts and reduce flare-ups.

The Alkaline Diet for Autoimmunity

The Alkaline diet is designed specifically to combat inflammatory diseases. You have to stick to the dietary habits to guarantee their compliance with the recommended Alkaline diets. You have to follow this protocol over long periods for better performance. Furthermore, you should be well aware of the principle of avoiding certain foods, particularly at night-time. During digestion, the body finally burns the food, except that it happens in a gradual and regulated way. When the body burns food, they actually leave a trail of ash just as when one burns wood in a fireplace. As mentioned earlier, this ash can be alkaline, inert, or acidic. This ash can directly affect the acidity in the body. So, if one eats acidic ash things, it makes the body acidic. If you eat meals of alkaline ash, it makes the body alkaline. Neutral ash has no effects.

Acidic ash is believed to make one susceptible to sickness and injuries, while alkaline ash is considered protective. Through consuming more alkaline ingredients, you might be encouraged to alkalize the diet and improve nutrients. Relevant foods considered to be alkaline, acidic, or neutral are accessible. These amounts of pH are not defined in the resting state, nor how they move within the body. You will be surprised to learn that, with its acidic qualities, citrus is an alkaline food.

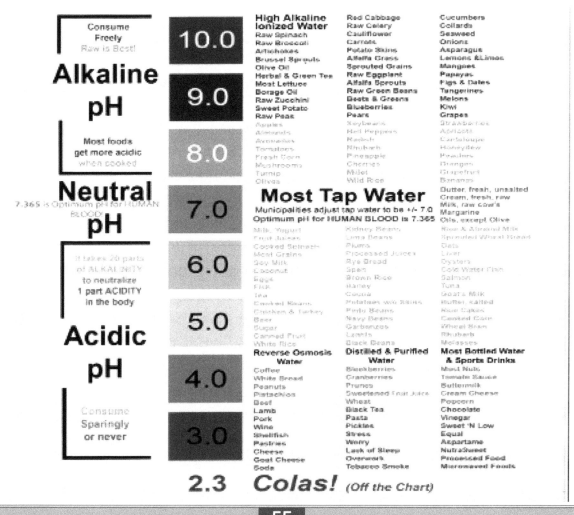

Certain food types are known to be alkaline, acidic, or neutral:

- Meat, livestock, seafood, food, eggs, alcohol, and grains are acidic.
- Starch, natural fats, and sugar are neutral.
- Fruits, nuts, legumes, and herbs are alkaline.

You should keep on with that as a life-changing diet, but not as a detox program. Through this diet, the intensity of your will and attention period will help you to extract the important benefits of lupus therapy. If you are more dedicated and stricter in your approach to this, you will find that all the recipes in this program will certainly have various advantages. You will find a significant increase in the inflammation that is caused by SLE. You will certainly love this concept since it is supported and can run for you. Foods with strong anti-inflammatory properties include fruits and vegetables, which are rich in compounds called antioxidants. Furthermore, foods such as fish, peanuts, ground flaxseed, canola oil, and omega-fatty acids containing olive oil can also aid battle inflammation. Saturated fats, on the other hand, can raise cholesterol levels. For patients with lupus, bone well-being is a specific issue. This is because therapies used to heal it will increase the risk of osteoporosis, a condition in which the bones grow less dense and easily break.

4.16 ALKALINE DIET AND OSTEOPOROSIS

A general theory of osteoporosis and nutrition is that the greater the acid load or acid out-put ability of the diet, the more a body has to work to retain a normal blood pH due to reduced kidney function, which in older people is known to be a much more important concern. The theory means that the body tries to guard against increasing acid by breaking down bone and muscle to obtain vital nutrients. Any researchers say that lots of fatty acids from Western diets may be a risk factor for osteoporosis. The acid load of a meal is determined not by the food's acidity after metabolism or by what the food produces during metabolism into the blood. Carbohydrates like slices of bread, cereals, rice, and noodles, as well as fish, meat, egg yolks, and cheeses, release acids into the bloodstream during metabolism. Vegetables and fruit break down to help neutralize the acid in order to add alkali to the body. There is no reason to remove items with higher acid loads from the diet, but they need to be consumed in abundance and properly combined with alkaline foods, so the net effect is a more alkaline, bone-healthy diet. Evidence shows that the best way to reduce dietary acid load is to eat lots of fruits and vegetables with minimal amounts of bread, cereals, and pasta, and good nutrients, but not excessive animal protein. Osteoporosis is a major risk factor for bone fractures, especially in females and older people. The amount of calcium lost in the urine is decreased by the Alkaline diet, lowering the risk of osteoporosis. The health of the skeleton is improved by eating more fruits and vegetables. Alkaline diets are abundant in these components.

Osteoporosis is a persistent bone disease characterized by a reduction in bone mineral content. It is highly popular among postmenopausal women and can dramatically increase the risk of fractures. In order to maintain a steady blood pH, most supporters of Alkaline diets say that the body gets alkaline minerals like calcium from the bones to counteract the acids from the acid-forming foods you eat. According to this theory, acid-forming foods, such as the conventional Western diet, will cause a drop in bone mineral density. This idea is known as the "hypothesis of osteoporosis acid-ash." Keep in mind that there are contradictory study data linking dietary acid with the bone structure or fracture probability. While no connection has been noted in much observational research, a substantial link has been identified by others.

Alkaline diets encourage bone stability by calcium retention and activating the IGF-1 receptor, which stimulates muscle and bone recovery.
In order to improve the bones, you might have discovered that you should consume more vegetables and fruit and eat less protein. This is how certain people believe that acidity in the body can be caused by protein-rich diets and weaken the bones.
Unfortunately, elevated acidity enhances the activity of the osteoclast, enhancing the risk of osteoporosis. Still, if the food does not lead to the acid residue, there is little need for the bones to give calcium. So, an increase of vegetables and fruits, with their alkaline residue, is ideal for bone structure. The body helps to neutralize the acidity of the blood by drawing calcium out of the muscles. Calcium is an alkaline earth metal, which neutralizes excess water. This might, probably, cause the bones to lose power.

How Does Alkaline Diet Help You Treat Osteoporosis?

People who accept the theory encourage the usage of the diet to impact the pH (acidity level) in the bloodstream, so the body does not need to absorb calcium from bones. This is regarded as an Alkaline diet. When consuming an Alkaline diet, one maximizes the intake of vegetables and fruit and lower the amount of protein from commodities like meat, dairy, and wheat. It is correct that the desire to eat loads of fruits and vegetables in the body has an alkaline influence that can help balance acid-forming foods. Vegetables and fruit can strengthen the muscles. Vitamin D and Calcium are what we need in order to prevent osteoporosis. We do require certain nutrients, of course, but there are other determinants of bone health than just intake of calcium and vitamin D. It is the overall consistency of the diet, which counts. For starters, hip fractures are higher in countries that consume milk. Since milk products are an outstanding source of calcium, it can be a surprise. So how is it that Asian-Americans are less vulnerable, with lower calcium intake, to osteoporosis? Not only does it contain the quantity of calcium or vitamin D, but it is the total content of the food that matters. The diet's acid-base balance seems to be a significant feature. This, though, is not entirely what people will think; acid is different because what you are thinking is on soda pop, vinegar, or fruit juice. Think of the base, and baking soda could jump into your brain. What matters, though, is not the alkalinity or acidity of the foods or liquids that one will consume but what happens to their components during digestion and metabolism. Proteins contain sulfur, acid is created from the foods consuming an immense amount of protein, and the sulfur is eventually converted within the body into sulfuric acid. As a consequence, acidic animals include fish, milk, poultry, and meat. Cereals and bread are also metabolized into acids. However, oddly, citrus foods do not contain acids. That's how citric acid in the body is broken into non-acidic elements. Although lentils and corn are acid-forming, the body retains an alkaline trace in most vegetables and fruits.

What does the strength of a bone have to do with this information? Providing a healthy acid-base balance is vital for health, and it is well understood that a body requires the surrounding fluid cells to be maintained at a pH between 7.35 to 7.45. Even the body will take steps to make sure that the pH of the extracellular fluid does not drop below 7.35, whether a meal is consumed with acid trace.

Kidneys can metabolize extra acid, carbon dioxide exhalation also enhances pH, and bones can release alkaline calcium salts to neutralize excess acid. The bone is complicated. There are always osteoblasts. Some osteoclasts are broken down. Unfortunately, elevated acidity enhances the activity of the osteoclast, enhancing the risk of osteoporosis. Researches have shown that carotenoids like beta carotene, lutein xanthan, and lycopene can improve bone density, as is found in many vegetables and fruits, but the cause for this is not clear.

4.17 BETTER HAIR HEALTH WITH ALKALINE DIET

When worrying about hair grooming, you can take the "if one goes slow, then one can go far" approach. It takes time for hair to reflect the affection and energy you invest in it, whether by fostering proper blood flow to the scalp or supplying the required nutrients for the body. In nutrition for hair growth, a safe approach, and lasting results are paramount. Hair growth is a long-term journey, and the results you will get would often be short-lived if you are searching for quick fixes and tricks. Fixing is not transforming. Transformation is directed at surviving. For those eager to accept a stand for their well-being and specifically hair well-being, they must take on an on-going commitment to cultivating healthy hair and restoring hair growth.

Our bodies are usually alkaline, meaning that the pH is roughly above 7, mostly on a pH scale of 0-14. When you modify the pH by consuming highly acidic foods, such as simple grains, alcohol, and refined meats, you change the environment in the body to become more acidic. The defensive mechanism, also known as inflammation, is turned on by the body to preserve the alkaline environment. In the comfort time, centered on simple intake and diseases, we are able to consume a handful of vitamins. And while it's one thing you can do to dramatically reduce inflammation in the body, we are unable to swap basic sugars with refined carbs. It has been shown again and again that sugar leads to inflammation that causes the bodies to enter their cells, including the hair follicles. And, there is an unconstructive belief that a couple of vitamins will cure their hair issues without changes to the diet.

One Diet Change Towards Hair Health

If you are about to create one shift in the diet, let it be cut out the sugar consumption to invest in hair growth and hair quality. If you can only accomplish one thing: say that by excluding white meal flour items, you can reach their hair growth targets: pasta and bread. It takes time to adapt, to there be no hurry in the on-going progress to improve oneself. The alkaline foods that are most common are:

- Leafy greens, spinach, kale, and broccoli.
- Avocado, raw (other than peanuts) almonds, and peas.
- Cucumber, celery, and cauliflower.

Another value of Alkaline diets is because it provides a greater concentration of fiber, leading to better food and healthier bowel movement. That you are not chronically bloated or constipated, not only "feel" nice for a balanced colon: because the intestines absorb the nutrients from foods, it is important to ensure that the nutrients from the diet reach the rest of the body. That includes certain nutrients that are vital to hair growth. To give the body an extra shot of alkalinity, one may even execute multiple hacks for the smoothies, such as adding wheatgrass and spirulina. However, it is important to ensure that you do not eat too much acidic stuff, such as:

- Sugar: White, wholemeal flour, baked goods, cakes, and pastries.
- Meat: Processed deli meats, fish, and poultry.
- Drinks: Black tea, coffee, alcohol, and fizzy/pop soda drinks.
- Dairy: Milk cheese of the least acidic dairy (goat cheese and cottage cheese are the less acidic option).

If you are frightened on the previous page to see all of the items you eat, here is another handy guide that separates the more and less acidic foods:

- Most acidic: Pop soda, alcohol, poultry, white, and wholemeal flour; meat and baked goods.
- Less acidic: Dairy, milk, fish, eggs, dark chocolate.

Reference on Meat and Milk

If you follow a plant-based diet, you can skip this portion. However, if you follow an omnivorous or vegetarian approach to eating and yet choose to ingest meat or dairy, you need to consume these, following the required amount of alkaline foods.

Food Conclusion for Growing Hair

It seems that when it comes to eating, everybody understands that they can eat less sugar and processed ingredients, everybody knows that too much of anything is awful for you, but maybe more of us can encourage healthy and balanced recipes to feed the bodies by thinking of everything from the point of view of "what's good for my hair." The hair would not expand dramatically if you eat a kale stalk each day for a week and even it out with a sugar binge over the weekend. It did not grow significantly after a week of living "healthily" without the sugar spree. In fact, it will not, even after a month of doing so. However, after a month, one might note a slight improvement in the energy levels: you notice that you have more energy, and you are more likely to add extra physical activity into the day, thereby improving your blood flow. You may have noticed that the hair looks better a little more than it used to after two months. After three months, you might see new hair development, especially if you mix it with stimulation of the scalp. They're small motions, so if you want to go high, you need to go steady.

Perfect Alkaline Diet to Prevent Hair-Loss

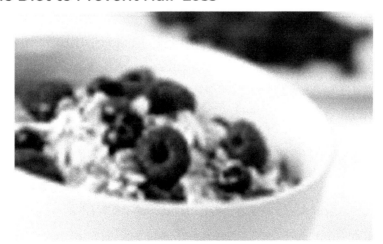

If you are getting a big hairline and bald spot, you are granted sleepless nights.

Here are some lifestyle improvements to maintain the mane better. Men are as sensitive as hair as females are with their hair. It's a delicate topic, one that raises many questions and leads to dramatic measures and paranoid treatments. However, because of the lather and rinse technique, no emphasis is put on nourishing hair until the problem begins. Before you begin losing sleep over baldness and book consultations with trichologists, take a closer look at what you're eating. The chances are that by incorporating ingredients that support hair growth and well-being, even small improvements made to what you eat will have a drastic impact. While genes and lifestyle may always have the upper hand, to better curb the hairline that is fading, here's what you can eat:

Carrots
Vitamin A-rich carrots, not just the hair, provide excellent nourishment for the scalp. A healthy scalp ensures shiny, well-conditioned hair that is improved and moisturized. Its decent diet of vegetables, lean proteins, and fruits, whole grains, fatty fish, legumes, Indian salmon, and low-fat milk are good promoters for healthier hair.

Prunes
The culprit could be depleting iron reserves if the hair suffers from thinning, dryness, exhaustion, discoloration, or falling hair. Prunes are proven to be outstanding sources of iron and help to significantly increase hair quality. Ensure you have plenty of green veggies and beetroots in the diet in addition to the prunes.

Green Peas
Although green peas are not rich in antioxidants or any particular vitamin or mineral, a well-balanced amount contains minerals and vitamins like iron, zinc, and B vitamins. This is important for healthy hair preservation.

Oats
Oats are packed with fiber to help preserve a healthy core and gut care. They also contain a wide concentration of other important nutrients, like iron, zinc, and Omega-6 fatty acids. They are all known as Polyunsaturated Fatty Acids (PUFAs). Omega-6 fatty acids, in general, are essential for the maintenance of normal skin, hair growth, and production. Since this essential ingredient is only

obtained from the diet, make sure the breakfast includes a bowl of oatmeal a few days of the week.

Shrimps

Although red meats are best stopped in excess, seeking an acceptable substitute for proteins may be a little challenging for those attempting to build muscle. Shrimps, instead, are a great addition to the vast variety of available seafood. They go very well in pasta and curry. They have all the nutrients needed to prevent hair-loss with their high concentration of vitamin B12, zinc, and iron.

Walnuts

Walnuts, not to be eclipsed by almonds, are one of the most skin and hair-friendly nuts in the group. In addition to containing more omega-6 fatty acids than any other food, walnuts often produce a great deal of iron, B vitamins (B1, zinc, B6, and B9), and a great deal of protein. These Walnuts, though, also contain a small residue of selenium, a mineral that is known to induce hair-loss in people that are selenium-deficient or have too much notice in their environment. So a few nuts will tide you over during the week without much trouble.

Eggs

With a head full of healthy hair, an egg is certainly one of the best friends. Vast numbers of essential nutrients such as vitamin B12, proteins, iron, Omega-6 fatty acids, and zinc, are filled up. It is recognized that being deficient in any of these minerals and vitamins results in low hair quality. Also, it is a good source of biotin (vitamin B7), a significant aid in the prevention of hair loss.

4.18 ALKALINE DIET AND KIDNEY DISEASES

The kidneys help regulate the blood pH level (acid intensity) by reducing excessive substances that can make the blood more alkaline and acidic. Blood that has a poor degree of pH is considered acidic and can cause life-threatening health problems. Expelling acid into the blood when one has a renal disease is more difficult for the kidneys. Because of this, one that is low in acidic, a High-Alkaline diet ingredient will allow people with kidney disease to manage their pH levels. In some cases, the doctor might order medication to assist with this balance. The food you consume will have an effect on the level of acid in the blood. Acid-contributing foods have a pH range of 0 to 7, whereas alkaline foods have a pH of 7 to 14.

- Fruits (if one is on a low-potassium diet).
- Others low-potassium are legumes.
- Textured soy protein.
- Egg whites.
- Vegetables.
- Eat fresh vegetables and fruits.

With more vegetables and fruits, a High-Alkaline diet can be a better way to help balance the pH levels. Usually, people with early kidney disease may not need to minimize potassium, so including more vegetables and fruits in their diet is not an issue. Individuals with late-stage kidney disease, though, still need to limit their potassium intake. It is easier to balance pH levels to keep potassium levels low, even low-potassium vegetables and fruit, for that purpose.

Scientific Evidence

The kidneys make bicarbonate ions that neutralize acids in your blood. Patients with Chronic Kidney Disorder (CKD) also have metabolic acidosis, that the kidney can no longer neutralize the acid load. Alkaline diets based on vegetables and fruits and mostly on plant protein may have a positive effect on long-term maintenance of renal function while retaining nutrient intake in patients with stage 4-5 CKD. Chronic Kidney Disease (CKD) is followed by a reduced propensity for acid excretion that has detrimental effects on acid-base, cardiovascular disease, and bone balance. The metabolic product, depending on the food form, may be neutral, acidic, or alkaline. The latest studies suggest that the intake of fiber-rich food typically improves renal impairment and disease growth. In people with symptomatic renal injury after treatment, there is a strong correlation between long-term preservation and alkaline dieting of renal function.

The kidney is used to regulate blood pH, but if kidney function declines and other tissues are metabolized to sustain pH, it is very likely that tissues may be saved, and Chronic Kidney Disease results may be improved by changing the diet to minimize the acid load. For instance, amino acid metabolism, after all, produces hydrogen ions, whereas vegetables and fruit produce organic salts that normally reduce the acid load when metabolized.

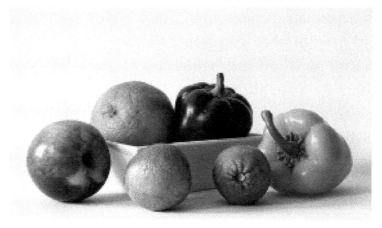

Lately, this hypothesis is being confirmed by a growing array of human trials utilizing vegetables and fruit and sodium bicarbonate to influence diet acid load. The first randomized clinical study on bicarbonate intake and CKD progression was performed by Ione de Brito-Ashurst and colleagues in 2009. There is bicarbonate in the kidneys, and it tends to neutralize the acid. In cases of Chronic Kidney Disease, 1-year bicarbonate supplementation slowed down the progression of kidney disease, as shown by creatinine clearance, and minimized the need for dialysis. The following year, in 2010, Donald Wesson's group published a five-year study, which reported a slow kidney failure as measured by bicarbonate supplementation's estimated Glomerular Filtration Rate (eGFR). Any later research by his group utilized bicarbonate or vegetables and fruits in order to achieve positive results. Goraya's research provided oral bicarbonate or acceptable vegetables and fruits that were reported to reduce the nutritional acid load by 50% for 30 days in Chronic Kidney patients and also recorded a slow decrease in eGFR at moderate but not mild amounts of disease in patients. In individuals with more progressed stages of CKD, 1-year of bicarbonate or vegetables and fruits did not prolong the decrease in eGFR, although certain urinary markers of kidney damage were minimized. Their most recent trial investigated whether kidney function may be maintained by reducing angiotensin II in transitional-stage CKD patients.

The decline in eGFR with bicarbonate or grown vegetables and fruits for three years and culminated in a similar decrease in the angiotensin II marker.

Many bicarbonate experiments from 6 months to 2 years have offered strong confirmation that acid load reduction consistently slows down eGFR degradation and improves indicators of bone health and muscle activity. All of the studies mentioned offered vegetables and fruit to patients free of charge to enhance adherence. It will be necessary to measure whether adherence can be maintained by education alone. In contrast, in optimizing efficiency and decreasing health care costs, "prescribing" vegetables and fruit may be more successful than bicarbonate, as both reduce blood pressure. There is accumulating data that, as dietary alkali, vegetables and fruits possibly aid in kidney failure.

4.19 THE BOTTOM LINE

While minimizing processed junk foods, an Alkaline diet is very healthy, facilitating a broad intake of bananas, vegetables, and sustainable plant foods. The Alkaline diet promotes health because of its alkalizing effects. Primarily, a low-protein alkalizing diet may help individuals with Chronic Kidney Disease. The Alkaline diet is generally healthier because it relies on fresh and unprocessed products. Consuming an Alkaline diet is important for the selection of vegetables and fruits over higher-calorie, higher-fat options. You may also avoid refined foods that often include a boatload of salt. Since these steps improve cholesterol and blood pressure reduction, which are both risk factors for cardiac failure, that's excellent news for cardiovascular health. To maintain a healthy weight, it is also important to avoid and control diabetes and osteoporosis. Some of the foods that are perfect for nourishing the body on the inside still render the body looks great on the outside. The health risks of living an alkaline lifestyle go well beyond hair, nails, and skin. You can have the naturally smooth, beautiful hair, and flawless, blemish-free skin that you need, and you can slow down the symptoms of the body's premature aging by feeding on an Alkaline diet.

It Will Makes Your Skin Glow

There is one popular equation, whether you suffer from rosacea, eczema, acne, psoriasis, or wrinkled skin. These skin disorders are concerns with acid. Your skin is the "third kidney," the primary organ of the body, and is an important organ for the body's purification. For detoxification, you have four main mechanisms: transpiration, urination, breathing, and defecation. Again, if you see something come up on your face, it's an indicator that the body is acidic and that the body is trying to hold the acids out like crazy. When you see the symptoms and results showing themselves on your face, it's time for alkalization.

You'll Have Stamina All Day Long

Your energy is an excellent predictor of how excellent you are in reality. Whenever one feels drained, one of the first things they can truly think of is water. A decrease in the hydration rate of only 5% will reduce up to 30% of your energy. As the average person loses 2.5 liters of water each day, it is recommended that one aim drink 3-4 liters of purified water per day, ideally at a pH of 8-9.5. To make the water more alkaline, introduce an edible lime or lemon slice, a spray of citrus, or supercharge the water with a scoop of Alkaline Standard Green.

You Will Sleep More Peacefully and Wake Up Refreshed

A tell-tale sign that you are acidic and maybe hoping for any help from the liver and the kidneys, your main detoxification organs, is waking up regularly between 1:00 to 3:00 am. The body is also the most toxic in the middle of the night, and if you do not routinely alkalize the body, the acid will keep you awake and prevent you from getting a night of healthy, deep REM sleep. Focus solely on dark green leafy vegetables during the day, such as kale, Swiss chard, watercress, and spinach, as well as wheatgrass, to help the body gradually detoxify the liver. Make sure to eat at least three hours before going to bed and reduce Acidic diets high in sugar and starch. Finally, potassium, calcium, magnesium, and sodium bicarbonates are very stimulating minerals in the nervous system and the most active acid neutralizer. Get up to thirty minutes of sleep, and that would be a game-changer!

You're Going to Have Good Teeth & Gums

Much when the body extracts calcium from the bones to neutralize acid, it can also steal nutrients from the teeth. Although in the teeth, there is just a small supply of nutrients, so any mineral deficiency can quickly contribute to the deterioration of the tooth and gum. It is important to reduce acid-high foods such as wheat, starch, and processed foods producing mouth-corroding acid. Finally, if you're dealing with an issue with gum or teeth, consider using coconut oil. Take 1-2 teaspoons. Actually, any toxins and bacteria in the mouth will "take" the oil away, increasing the well-being of the mouth.

Conclusion

Alfredo Bowman was a healer and herbalist best known as Dr. Sebi. He, a pathologist, and naturalist, spent decades researching the plants and herbs of Africa, the Caribbean, North, South, and Central America. In that experience, his unique approach to curing the human body is deeply embedded.

It diametrically contradicts the present Western strategy as we explore an African approach to disease. The African Bio-Mineral Balance, precisely, refutes the premise of germ/virus/bacteria. A study by Dr. Sebi shows that any disease manifestation discovers its origin where and when the mucous membrane has been damaged. For instance, if there is excess mucous membrane in the bronchial passages, bronchitis is the disease; if it is in the lungs, pneumonia is the disease; diabetes if it is in the pancreatic duct; arthritis if it is in the joints. Both African Bio-Mineral Balance compounds compose of natural plants, indicating that their composition is alkaline in nature. Each cell in the body can be cleaned with Dr. Sebi's intracellular detoxifying washing technique and diet. Then the body will regenerate, and there will be rejuvenation. Bio-Mineral Treatment, which is a natural food for vegetation cells, is provided by Dr. Sebi. In essence, it is a living substance which at the cellular level, nourishes the body and detoxifies.

As recommended by Dr. Sebi, the Alkaline diet meal plans rely on the approved ingredients contained in the dietary guidelines of the diet. With limited quantities of the other food classes, meals on the plan prioritize salads and fruits. The diet of Dr. Sebi encourages consuming whole, unprocessed food focused on plants. If you do not usually in your daily life, it may support weight-loss. The diet of Dr. Sebi stresses the intake of nutrient-rich foods, fruits, whole grains, and good fats that can minimize the risk of heart disease, stroke, osteoporosis, lupus, diabetes, herpes, tuberculosis, and inflammation.

Lightning Source UK Ltd.
Milton Keynes UK
UKHW050652120321
380219UK00002B/112